Housekeeping

Belong to _____

Cleaning Checklist

Month:

Kitchen:
- ○ Wash and put away dishes
- ○ Wipe down cabinets
- ○ Organize cabinets
- ○ Organize pantry items
- ○ Empty trash
- ○ Scrub inside of microwave
- ○ Deep clean oven & stovetop
- ○ Scrub & disinfect sink
- ○ Clean all appliances
- ○ Wash out garbage can
- ○ Broken or Incomplete dishes

Bathrooms:
- ○ Clean/wash shower curtain
- ○ Wipe down mirrors
- ○ Wash out trash can
- ○ Scrub toilet
- ○ Empty trash
- ○ Scrub bathtub & faucet
- ○ Clean out/organize cabinets
- ○ Scrub shower walls & fixtures
- ○ Wipe down cabinets

Living room:
- ○ Dust electronics
- ○ Dust mantel/shelves
- ○ Steam clean chairs
- ○ Dust tabletops
- ○ Organize media cabinet

Bedrooms:
- ○ Wash bedding
- ○ Wash pillows
- ○ Pick up clothes
- ○ Vacuum & clean window sills
- ○ Dust light fixtures & fans
- ○ Wash windows

Weekly Cleaning Checklist

Week:

Complete tasks daily

MONDAY

TUESDAY

WEDNESDAY

THURDAY

FRIDAY

SATURDAY

SUNDAY

NOTE

Weekly Cleaning Checklist

Week:

Complete tasks daily

MONDAY

TUESDAY

WEDNESDAY

THURDAY

FRIDAY

SATURDAY

SUNDAY

NOTE

Weekly Cleaning Checklist

Week:

Complete tasks daily

MONDAY

TUESDAY

WEDNESDAY

THURDAY

FRIDAY

SATURDAY

SUNDAY

NOTE

Weekly Cleaning Checklist

Week:

Complete tasks daily

MONDAY

TUESDAY

WEDNESDAY

THURDAY

FRIDAY

SATURDAY

SUNDAY

NOTE

Cleaning Checklist

Month:

Kitchen:
- ○ Wash and put away dishes
- ○ Wipe down cabinets
- ○ Organize cabinets
- ○ Organize pantry items
- ○ Empty trash
- ○ Scrub inside of microwave
- ○ Deep clean oven & stovetop
- ○ Scrub & disinfect sink
- ○ Clean all appliances
- ○ Wash out garbage can
- ○ Broken or Incomplete dishes
- ○
- ○
- ○
- ○
- ○

Bathrooms:
- ○ Clean/wash shower curtain
- ○ Wipe down mirrors
- ○ Wash out trash can
- ○ Scrub toilet
- ○ Empty trash
- ○ Scrub bathtub & faucet
- ○ Clean out/organize cabinets
- ○ Scrub shower walls & fixtures
- ○ Wipe down cabinets
- ○
- ○
- ○
- ○
- ○
- ○
- ○

Living room:
- ○ Dust electronics
- ○ Dust mantel/shelves
- ○ Steam clean chairs
- ○ Dust tabletops
- ○ Organize media cabinet
- ○
- ○
- ○
- ○
- ○
- ○
- ○
- ○
- ○
- ○
- ○

Bedrooms:
- ○ Wash bedding
- ○ Wash pillows
- ○ Pick up clothes
- ○ Vacuum & clean window sills
- ○ Dust light fixtures & fans
- ○ Wash windows
- ○
- ○
- ○
- ○
- ○
- ○
- ○
- ○
- ○
- ○

Weekly Cleaning Checklist

Week:

Complete tasks daily

MONDAY

TUESDAY

WEDNESDAY

THURSDAY

FRIDAY

SATURDAY

SUNDAY

NOTE

Weekly Cleaning Checklist

Week:

Complete tasks daily

MONDAY

TUESDAY

WEDNESDAY

THURSDAY

FRIDAY

SATURDAY

SUNDAY

NOTE

Weekly Cleaning Checklist

Week:

Complete tasks daily

MONDAY

TUESDAY

WEDNESDAY

THURDAY

FRIDAY

SATURDAY

SUNDAY

NOTE

Weekly Cleaning Checklist

Week:

Complete tasks daily

MONDAY

TUESDAY

WEDNESDAY

THURSDAY

FRIDAY

SATURDAY

SUNDAY

NOTE

Cleaning Checklist

Month:

Kitchen:
- ○ Wash and put away dishes
- ○ Wipe down cabinets
- ○ Organize cabinets
- ○ Organize pantry items
- ○ Empty trash
- ○ Scrub inside of microwave
- ○ Deep clean oven & stovetop
- ○ Scrub & disinfect sink
- ○ Clean all appliances
- ○ Wash out garbage can
- ○ Broken or Incomplete dishes

Bathrooms:
- ○ Clean/wash shower curtain
- ○ Wipe down mirrors
- ○ Wash out trash can
- ○ Scrub toilet
- ○ Empty trash
- ○ Scrub bathtub & faucet
- ○ Clean out/organize cabinets
- ○ Scrub shower walls & fixtures
- ○ Wipe down cabinets

Living room:
- ○ Dust electronics
- ○ Dust mantel/shelves
- ○ Steam clean chairs
- ○ Dust tabletops
- ○ Organize media cabinet

Bedrooms:
- ○ Wash bedding
- ○ Wash pillows
- ○ Pick up clothes
- ○ Vacuum & clean window sills
- ○ Dust light fixtures & fans
- ○ Wash windows

Weekly Cleaning Checklist

Week:

Complete tasks daily

MONDAY

TUESDAY

WEDNESDAY

THURDAY

FRIDAY

SATURDAY

SUNDAY

NOTE

Weekly Cleaning Checklist

Week:

Complete tasks daily

MONDAY

TUESDAY

WEDNESDAY

THURSDAY

FRIDAY

SATURDAY

SUNDAY

NOTE

Weekly Cleaning Checklist

Week:

Complete tasks daily

MONDAY

TUESDAY

WEDNESDAY

THURDAY

FRIDAY

SATURDAY

SUNDAY

NOTE

Weekly Cleaning Checklist

Week:

Complete tasks daily

MONDAY

TUESDAY

WEDNESDAY

THURDAY

FRIDAY

SATURDAY

SUNDAY

NOTE

Cleaning Checklist

Month:

Kitchen:
- ◯ Wash and put away dishes
- ◯ Wipe down cabinets
- ◯ Organize cabinets
- ◯ Organize pantry items
- ◯ Empty trash
- ◯ Scrub inside of microwave
- ◯ Deep clean oven & stovetop
- ◯ Scrub & disinfect sink
- ◯ Clean all appliances
- ◯ Wash out garbage can
- ◯ Broken or Incomplete dishes

Bathrooms:
- ◯ Clean/wash shower curtain
- ◯ Wipe down mirrors
- ◯ Wash out trash can
- ◯ Scrub toilet
- ◯ Empty trash
- ◯ Scrub bathtub & faucet
- ◯ Clean out/organize cabinets
- ◯ Scrub shower walls & fixtures
- ◯ Wipe down cabinets

Living room:
- ◯ Dust electronics
- ◯ Dust mantel/shelves
- ◯ Steam clean chairs
- ◯ Dust tabletops
- ◯ Organize media cabinet

Bedrooms:
- ◯ Wash bedding
- ◯ Wash pillows
- ◯ Pick up clothes
- ◯ Vacuum & clean window sills
- ◯ Dust light fixtures & fans
- ◯ Wash windows

Weekly Cleaning Checklist

Week:

Complete tasks daily

MONDAY

TUESDAY

WEDNESDAY

THURSDAY

FRIDAY

SATURDAY

SUNDAY

NOTE

Weekly Cleaning Checklist

Week:

Complete tasks daily

MONDAY

TUESDAY

WEDNESDAY

THURDAY

FRIDAY

SATURDAY

SUNDAY

NOTE

Weekly Cleaning Checklist

Week:

Complete tasks daily

MONDAY

TUESDAY

WEDNESDAY

THURDAY

FRIDAY

SATURDAY

SUNDAY

NOTE

Weekly Cleaning Checklist

Week:

Complete tasks daily

MONDAY

TUESDAY

WEDNESDAY

THURSDAY

FRIDAY

SATURDAY

SUNDAY

NOTE

Cleaning Checklist

Month:

Kitchen:
- ☐ Wash and put away dishes
- ☐ Wipe down cabinets
- ☐ Organize cabinets
- ☐ Organize pantry items
- ☐ Empty trash
- ☐ Scrub inside of microwave
- ☐ Deep clean oven & stovetop
- ☐ Scrub & disinfect sink
- ☐ Clean all appliances
- ☐ Wash out garbage can
- ☐ Broken or Incomplete dishes

Bathrooms:
- ☐ Clean/wash shower curtain
- ☐ Wipe down mirrors
- ☐ Wash out trash can
- ☐ Scrub toilet
- ☐ Empty trash
- ☐ Scrub bathtub & faucet
- ☐ Clean out/organize cabinets
- ☐ Scrub shower walls & fixtures
- ☐ Wipe down cabinets

Living room:
- ☐ Dust electronics
- ☐ Dust mantel/shelves
- ☐ Steam clean chairs
- ☐ Dust tabletops
- ☐ Organize media cabinet

Bedrooms:
- ☐ Wash bedding
- ☐ Wash pillows
- ☐ Pick up clothes
- ☐ Vacuum & clean window sills
- ☐ Dust light fixtures & fans
- ☐ Wash windows

Weekly Cleaning Checklist

Week:

Complete tasks daily

MONDAY

TUESDAY

WEDNESDAY

THURDAY

FRIDAY

SATURDAY

SUNDAY

NOTE

Weekly Cleaning Checklist

Week:

Complete tasks daily

MONDAY

TUESDAY

WEDNESDAY

THURDAY

FRIDAY

SATURDAY

SUNDAY

NOTE

Weekly Cleaning Checklist

Week:

Complete tasks daily

MONDAY

TUESDAY

WEDNESDAY

THURDAY

FRIDAY

SATURDAY

SUNDAY

NOTE

Weekly Cleaning Checklist

Week:

Complete tasks daily

MONDAY

TUESDAY

WEDNESDAY

THURDAY

FRIDAY

SATURDAY

SUNDAY

NOTE

Cleaning Checklist

Month:

Kitchen:
- ○ Wash and put away dishes
- ○ Wipe down cabinets
- ○ Organize cabinets
- ○ Organize pantry items
- ○ Empty trash
- ○ Scrub inside of microwave
- ○ Deep clean oven & stovetop
- ○ Scrub & disinfect sink
- ○ Clean all appliances
- ○ Wash out garbage can
- ○ Broken or Incomplete dishes

Bathrooms:
- ○ Clean/wash shower curtain
- ○ Wipe down mirrors
- ○ Wash out trash can
- ○ Scrub toilet
- ○ Empty trash
- ○ Scrub bathtub & faucet
- ○ Clean out/organize cabinets
- ○ Scrub shower walls & fixtures
- ○ Wipe down cabinets

Living room:
- ○ Dust electronics
- ○ Dust mantel/shelves
- ○ Steam clean chairs
- ○ Dust tabletops
- ○ Organize media cabinet

Bedrooms:
- ○ Wash bedding
- ○ Wash pillows
- ○ Pick up clothes
- ○ Vacuum & clean window sills
- ○ Dust light fixtures & fans
- ○ Wash windows

Weekly Cleaning Checklist

Week:

Complete tasks daily

MONDAY

TUESDAY

WEDNESDAY

THURDAY

FRIDAY

SATURDAY

SUNDAY

NOTE

Weekly Cleaning Checklist

Week:

Complete tasks daily

MONDAY

TUESDAY

WEDNESDAY

THURDAY

FRIDAY

SATURDAY

SUNDAY

NOTE

Weekly Cleaning Checklist

Week:

Complete tasks daily

MONDAY

TUESDAY

WEDNESDAY

THURDAY

FRIDAY

SATURDAY

SUNDAY

NOTE

Weekly Cleaning Checklist

Week:

Complete tasks daily

MONDAY

TUESDAY

WEDNESDAY

THURSDAY

FRIDAY

SATURDAY

SUNDAY

NOTE

Cleaning Checklist

Month:

Kitchen:
- ○ Wash and put away dishes
- ○ Wipe down cabinets
- ○ Organize cabinets
- ○ Organize pantry items
- ○ Empty trash
- ○ Scrub inside of microwave
- ○ Deep clean oven & stovetop
- ○ Scrub & disinfect sink
- ○ Clean all appliances
- ○ Wash out garbage can
- ○ Broken or Incomplete dishes

Bathrooms:
- ○ Clean/wash shower curtain
- ○ Wipe down mirrors
- ○ Wash out trash can
- ○ Scrub toilet
- ○ Empty trash
- ○ Scrub bathtub & faucet
- ○ Clean out/organize cabinets
- ○ Scrub shower walls & fixtures
- ○ Wipe down cabinets

Living room:
- ○ Dust electronics
- ○ Dust mantel/shelves
- ○ Steam clean chairs
- ○ Dust tabletops
- ○ Organize media cabinet

Bedrooms:
- ○ Wash bedding
- ○ Wash pillows
- ○ Pick up clothes
- ○ Vacuum & clean window sills
- ○ Dust light fixtures & fans
- ○ Wash windows

Weekly Cleaning Checklist

Week:

Complete tasks daily

MONDAY

TUESDAY

WEDNESDAY

THURDAY

FRIDAY

SATURDAY

SUNDAY

NOTE

Weekly Cleaning Checklist

Week:

Complete tasks daily

MONDAY

TUESDAY

WEDNESDAY

THURDAY

FRIDAY

SATURDAY

SUNDAY

NOTE

Weekly Cleaning Checklist

Week:

Complete tasks daily

MONDAY

TUESDAY

WEDNESDAY

THURDAY

FRIDAY

SATURDAY

SUNDAY

NOTE

Weekly Cleaning Checklist

Week:

Complete tasks daily

MONDAY

TUESDAY

WEDNESDAY

THURDAY

FRIDAY

SATURDAY

SUNDAY

NOTE

Cleaning Checklist

Month:

Kitchen:
- ◯ Wash and put away dishes
- ◯ Wipe down cabinets
- ◯ Organize cabinets
- ◯ Organize pantry items
- ◯ Empty trash
- ◯ Scrub inside of microwave
- ◯ Deep clean oven & stovetop
- ◯ Scrub & disinfect sink
- ◯ Clean all appliances
- ◯ Wash out garbage can
- ◯ Broken or Incomplete dishes

Bathrooms:
- ◯ Clean/wash shower curtain
- ◯ Wipe down mirrors
- ◯ Wash out trash can
- ◯ Scrub toilet
- ◯ Empty trash
- ◯ Scrub bathtub & faucet
- ◯ Clean out/organize cabinets
- ◯ Scrub shower walls & fixtures
- ◯ Wipe down cabinets

Living room:
- ◯ Dust electronics
- ◯ Dust mantel/shelves
- ◯ Steam clean chairs
- ◯ Dust tabletops
- ◯ Organize media cabinet

Bedrooms:
- ◯ Wash bedding
- ◯ Wash pillows
- ◯ Pick up clothes
- ◯ Vacuum & clean window sills
- ◯ Dust light fixtures & fans
- ◯ Wash windows

Weekly Cleaning Checklist

Week:

Complete tasks daily

MONDAY

TUESDAY

WEDNESDAY

THURSDAY

FRIDAY

SATURDAY

SUNDAY

NOTE

Weekly Cleaning Checklist

Week:

Complete tasks daily

MONDAY

TUESDAY

WEDNESDAY

THURDAY

FRIDAY

SATURDAY

SUNDAY

NOTE

Weekly Cleaning Checklist

Week:

Complete tasks daily

MONDAY

TUESDAY

WEDNESDAY

THURDAY

FRIDAY

SATURDAY

SUNDAY

NOTE

Weekly Cleaning Checklist

Week:

Complete tasks daily

MONDAY

TUESDAY

WEDNESDAY

THURDAY

FRIDAY

SATURDAY

SUNDAY

NOTE

Cleaning Checklist

Month:

Kitchen:
- ○ Wash and put away dishes
- ○ Wipe down cabinets
- ○ Organize cabinets
- ○ Organize pantry items
- ○ Empty trash
- ○ Scrub inside of microwave
- ○ Deep clean oven & stovetop
- ○ Scrub & disinfect sink
- ○ Clean all appliances
- ○ Wash out garbage can
- ○ Broken or Incomplete dishes

Bathrooms:
- ○ Clean/wash shower curtain
- ○ Wipe down mirrors
- ○ Wash out trash can
- ○ Scrub toilet
- ○ Empty trash
- ○ Scrub bathtub & faucet
- ○ Clean out/organize cabinets
- ○ Scrub shower walls & fixtures
- ○ Wipe down cabinets

Living room:
- ○ Dust electronics
- ○ Dust mantel/shelves
- ○ Steam clean chairs
- ○ Dust tabletops
- ○ Organize media cabinet

Bedrooms:
- ○ Wash bedding
- ○ Wash pillows
- ○ Pick up clothes
- ○ Vacuum & clean window sills
- ○ Dust light fixtures & fans
- ○ Wash windows

Weekly Cleaning Checklist

Week:

Complete tasks daily

MONDAY

TUESDAY

WEDNESDAY

THURDAY

FRIDAY

SATURDAY

SUNDAY

NOTE

Weekly Cleaning Checklist

Week:

Complete tasks daily

MONDAY

TUESDAY

WEDNESDAY

THURDAY

FRIDAY

SATURDAY

SUNDAY

NOTE

Weekly Cleaning Checklist

Week:

Complete tasks daily

MONDAY

TUESDAY

WEDNESDAY

THURDAY

FRIDAY

SATURDAY

SUNDAY

NOTE

Weekly Cleaning Checklist

Week:

Complete tasks daily

MONDAY

TUESDAY

WEDNESDAY

THURDAY

FRIDAY

SATURDAY

SUNDAY

NOTE

Cleaning Checklist

Month:

Kitchen:
- ○ Wash and put away dishes
- ○ Wipe down cabinets
- ○ Organize cabinets
- ○ Organize pantry items
- ○ Empty trash
- ○ Scrub inside of microwave
- ○ Deep clean oven & stovetop
- ○ Scrub & disinfect sink
- ○ Clean all appliances
- ○ Wash out garbage can
- ○ Broken or Incomplete dishes

Bathrooms:
- ○ Clean/wash shower curtain
- ○ Wipe down mirrors
- ○ Wash out trash can
- ○ Scrub toilet
- ○ Empty trash
- ○ Scrub bathtub & faucet
- ○ Clean out/organize cabinets
- ○ Scrub shower walls & fixtures
- ○ Wipe down cabinets

Living room:
- ○ Dust electronics
- ○ Dust mantel/shelves
- ○ Steam clean chairs
- ○ Dust tabletops
- ○ Organize media cabinet

Bedrooms:
- ○ Wash bedding
- ○ Wash pillows
- ○ Pick up clothes
- ○ Vacuum & clean window sills
- ○ Dust light fixtures & fans
- ○ Wash windows

Weekly Cleaning Checklist

Week:

Complete tasks daily

MONDAY

TUESDAY

WEDNESDAY

THURDAY

FRIDAY

SATURDAY

SUNDAY

NOTE

Weekly Cleaning Checklist

Week:

Complete tasks daily

MONDAY

TUESDAY

WEDNESDAY

THURDAY

FRIDAY

SATURDAY

SUNDAY

NOTE

Weekly Cleaning Checklist

Week:

Complete tasks daily

MONDAY

TUESDAY

WEDNESDAY

THURSDAY

FRIDAY

SATURDAY

SUNDAY

NOTE

Weekly Cleaning Checklist

Week:

Complete tasks daily

MONDAY

TUESDAY

WEDNESDAY

THURSDAY

FRIDAY

SATURDAY

SUNDAY

NOTE

Cleaning Checklist

Month:

Kitchen:
- ○ Wash and put away dishes
- ○ Wipe down cabinets
- ○ Organize cabinets
- ○ Organize pantry items
- ○ Empty trash
- ○ Scrub inside of microwave
- ○ Deep clean oven & stovetop
- ○ Scrub & disinfect sink
- ○ Clean all appliances
- ○ Wash out garbage can
- ○ Broken or Incomplete dishes

Bathrooms:
- ○ Clean/wash shower curtain
- ○ Wipe down mirrors
- ○ Wash out trash can
- ○ Scrub toilet
- ○ Empty trash
- ○ Scrub bathtub & faucet
- ○ Clean out/organize cabinets
- ○ Scrub shower walls & fixtures
- ○ Wipe down cabinets

Living room:
- ○ Dust electronics
- ○ Dust mantel/shelves
- ○ Steam clean chairs
- ○ Dust tabletops
- ○ Organize media cabinet

Bedrooms:
- ○ Wash bedding
- ○ Wash pillows
- ○ Pick up clothes
- ○ Vacuum & clean window sills
- ○ Dust light fixtures & fans
- ○ Wash windows

Weekly Cleaning Checklist

Week:

Complete tasks daily

MONDAY

TUESDAY

WEDNESDAY

THURDAY

FRIDAY

SATURDAY

SUNDAY

NOTE

Weekly Cleaning Checklist

Week:

Complete tasks daily

MONDAY

TUESDAY

WEDNESDAY

THURDAY

FRIDAY

SATURDAY

SUNDAY

NOTE

Weekly Cleaning Checklist

Week:

Complete tasks daily

MONDAY

TUESDAY

WEDNESDAY

THURDAY

FRIDAY

SATURDAY

SUNDAY

NOTE

Weekly Cleaning Checklist

Week:

Complete tasks daily

MONDAY

THURSDAY

TUESDAY

FRIDAY

WEDNESDAY

SATURDAY

SUNDAY

NOTE

Cleaning Checklist

Month:

Kitchen:
- ○ Wash and put away dishes
- ○ Wipe down cabinets
- ○ Organize cabinets
- ○ Organize pantry items
- ○ Empty trash
- ○ Scrub inside of microwave
- ○ Deep clean oven & stovetop
- ○ Scrub & disinfect sink
- ○ Clean all appliances
- ○ Wash out garbage can
- ○ Broken or Incomplete dishes

Bathrooms:
- ○ Clean/wash shower curtain
- ○ Wipe down mirrors
- ○ Wash out trash can
- ○ Scrub toilet
- ○ Empty trash
- ○ Scrub bathtub & faucet
- ○ Clean out/organize cabinets
- ○ Scrub shower walls & fixtures
- ○ Wipe down cabinets

Living room:
- ○ Dust electronics
- ○ Dust mantel/shelves
- ○ Steam clean chairs
- ○ Dust tabletops
- ○ Organize media cabinet

Bedrooms:
- ○ Wash bedding
- ○ Wash pillows
- ○ Pick up clothes
- ○ Vacuum & clean window sills
- ○ Dust light fixtures & fans
- ○ Wash windows

Weekly Cleaning Checklist

Week:

Complete tasks daily

- ○ ....
- ○ ....
- ○ ....
- ○ ....
- ○ ....
- ○ ....
- ○ ....
- ○ ....
- ○ ....

MONDAY
- ○ ....
- ○ ....
- ○ ....
- ○ ....
- ○ ....
- ○ ....

THURSDAY
- ○ ....
- ○ ....
- ○ ....
- ○ ....
- ○ ....
- ○ ....

TUESDAY
- ○ ....
- ○ ....
- ○ ....
- ○ ....
- ○ ....
- ○ ....

FRIDAY
- ○ ....
- ○ ....
- ○ ....
- ○ ....
- ○ ....
- ○ ....

WEDNESDAY
- ○ ....
- ○ ....
- ○ ....
- ○ ....
- ○ ....
- ○ ....

SATURDAY
- ○ ....
- ○ ....
- ○ ....
- ○ ....
- ○ ....
- ○ ....

SUNDAY
- ○ ....
- ○ ....
- ○ ....
- ○ ....
- ○ ....
- ○ ....

NOTE

Weekly Cleaning Checklist

Week:

Complete tasks daily

MONDAY

TUESDAY

WEDNESDAY

THURDAY

FRIDAY

SATURDAY

SUNDAY

NOTE

Weekly Cleaning Checklist

Week:

Complete tasks daily

MONDAY

TUESDAY

WEDNESDAY

THURDAY

FRIDAY

SATURDAY

SUNDAY

NOTE

Weekly Cleaning Checklist

Week:

Complete tasks daily

MONDAY

TUESDAY

WEDNESDAY

THURSDAY

FRIDAY

SATURDAY

SUNDAY

NOTE

Made in the USA
Monee, IL
14 May 2021